Blood Glucose Logbook

Copyright ©

All rights reserved.
No parts of this publication may be reproduced, distributed, or transmitted in any
form, or by any means, including photocopying, recording or other electronic or
mechanical methods, without prior written permission from the publisher.

Date ....

Sleep quality and duration ....

Stress levels   1   2   3   4   5   6   7   8   9   10

Water Intake   ▯ ▯ ▯ ▯ ▯ ▯ ▯ ▯ ▯ ▯

Time	Blood Glucose	Food Intake	Exercise

Medication   Symptoms   Notes
....
....
....
....
....

Date ....

Sleep quality and duration ....

Stress levels   1   2   3   4   5   6   7   8   9   10

Water Intake ⬜ ⬜ ⬜ ⬜ ⬜ ⬜ ⬜ ⬜ ⬜ ⬜

Time	Blood Glucose	Food Intake	Exercise

Medication   Symptoms   Notes
....
....
....
....
....

Date ....

Sleep quality and duration ....

Stress levels   1   2   3   4   5   6   7   8   9   10

Water Intake ▯ ▯ ▯ ▯ ▯ ▯ ▯ ▯ ▯ ▯

Time	Blood Glucose	Food Intake	Exercise

Medication   Symptoms   Notes
....
....
....
....
....

Date ....

Sleep quality and duration ....

Stress levels   1   2   3   4   5   6   7   8   9   10

Water Intake   ⬜ ⬜ ⬜ ⬜ ⬜ ⬜ ⬜ ⬜ ⬜ ⬜

Time	Blood Glucose	Food Intake	Exercise

Medication   Symptoms   Notes
....
....
....
....
....

Date ....

Sleep quality and duration ....

Stress levels   1   2   3   4   5   6   7   8   9   10

Water Intake   ▯ ▯ ▯ ▯ ▯ ▯ ▯ ▯ ▯ ▯

Time	Blood Glucose	Food Intake	Exercise

Medication   Symptoms   Notes

Date ....

Sleep quality and duration ....

Stress levels   1   2   3   4   5   6   7   8   9   10

Water Intake   ☐ ☐ ☐ ☐ ☐ ☐ ☐ ☐ ☐ ☐

Time	Blood Glucose	Food Intake	Exercise

Medication   Symptoms   Notes
....
....
....
....
....

Date ....

Sleep quality and duration ....

Stress levels   1   2   3   4   5   6   7   8   9   10

Water Intake   ⬜ ⬜ ⬜ ⬜ ⬜ ⬜ ⬜ ⬜ ⬜ ⬜

Time	Blood Glucose	Food Intake	Exercise

Medication   Symptoms   Notes
....
....
....
....
....

Date ....

Sleep quality and duration ....

Stress levels   1   2   3   4   5   6   7   8   9   10

Water Intake   ▯ ▯ ▯ ▯ ▯ ▯ ▯ ▯ ▯ ▯

Time	Blood Glucose	Food Intake	Exercise

Medication   Symptoms   Notes
....
....
....
....
....

Date ....

Sleep quality and duration ....

Stress levels   1   2   3   4   5   6   7   8   9   10

Water Intake   ▯ ▯ ▯ ▯ ▯ ▯ ▯ ▯ ▯ ▯

Time	Blood Glucose	Food Intake	Exercise

Medication   Symptoms   Notes
....
....
....
....
....

Date ....

Sleep quality and duration ....

Stress levels 1 2 3 4 5 6 7 8 9 10

Water Intake ⊔ ⊔ ⊔ ⊔ ⊔ ⊔ ⊔ ⊔ ⊔ ⊔

Time	Blood Glucose	Food Intake	Exercise

Medication   Symptoms   Notes
....
....
....
....
....

Date ....

Sleep quality and duration ....

Stress levels   1   2   3   4   5   6   7   8   9   10

Water Intake   ☐ ☐ ☐ ☐ ☐ ☐ ☐ ☐ ☐ ☐

Time	Blood Glucose	Food Intake	Exercise

Medication   Symptoms   Notes
....
....
....
....
....

Date ....

Sleep quality and duration ....

Stress levels   1   2   3   4   5   6   7   8   9   10

Water Intake ⌴ ⌴ ⌴ ⌴ ⌴ ⌴ ⌴ ⌴ ⌴ ⌴

Time	Blood Glucose	Food Intake	Exercise

Medication   Symptoms   Notes
....
....
....
....
....

Date ....

Sleep quality and duration ....

Stress levels   1   2   3   4   5   6   7   8   9   10

Water Intake   ▯ ▯ ▯ ▯ ▯ ▯ ▯ ▯ ▯ ▯

Time	Blood Glucose	Food Intake	Exercise

Medication   Symptoms   Notes
....
....
....
....
....

Date ....

Sleep quality and duration ....

Stress levels   1   2   3   4   5   6   7   8   9   10

Water Intake   ⬜ ⬜ ⬜ ⬜ ⬜ ⬜ ⬜ ⬜ ⬜ ⬜

Time	Blood Glucose	Food Intake	Exercise

Medication   Symptoms   Notes
....
....
....
....
....

Date ....

Sleep quality and duration ....

Stress levels   1   2   3   4   5   6   7   8   9   10

Water Intake   ▯ ▯ ▯ ▯ ▯ ▯ ▯ ▯ ▯ ▯

Time	Blood Glucose	Food Intake	Exercise

Medication   Symptoms   Notes
....
....
....
....
....

Date ....

Sleep quality and duration ....

Stress levels   1   2   3   4   5   6   7   8   9   10

Water Intake ▯ ▯ ▯ ▯ ▯ ▯ ▯ ▯ ▯ ▯

Time	Blood Glucose	Food Intake	Exercise

Medication   Symptoms   Notes
....
....
....
....
....

Date ....

Sleep quality and duration ....

Stress levels   1   2   3   4   5   6   7   8   9   10

Water Intake   ☐ ☐ ☐ ☐ ☐ ☐ ☐ ☐ ☐ ☐

Time	Blood Glucose	Food Intake	Exercise

Medication	Symptoms	Notes
....	....	....
....	....	....
....	....	....
....	....	....
....	....	....

Date ....

Sleep quality and duration ....

Stress levels   1   2   3   4   5   6   7   8   9   10

Water Intake ⬜ ⬜ ⬜ ⬜ ⬜ ⬜ ⬜ ⬜ ⬜ ⬜

Time	Blood Glucose	Food Intake	Exercise

Medication   Symptoms   Notes
....
....
....
....
....

Date ....

Sleep quality and duration ....

Stress levels   1   2   3   4   5   6   7   8   9   10

Water Intake   ▯ ▯ ▯ ▯ ▯ ▯ ▯ ▯ ▯ ▯

Time	Blood Glucose	Food Intake	Exercise

Medication   Symptoms   Notes
....
....
....
....
....

Date ....

Sleep quality and duration ....

Stress levels   1   2   3   4   5   6   7   8   9   10

Water Intake ▯ ▯ ▯ ▯ ▯ ▯ ▯ ▯ ▯ ▯

Time	Blood Glucose	Food Intake	Exercise

Medication   Symptoms   Notes
....
....
....
....
....

Date ....

Sleep quality and duration ....

Stress levels   1   2   3   4   5   6   7   8   9   10

Water Intake ▯ ▯ ▯ ▯ ▯ ▯ ▯ ▯ ▯ ▯

Time	Blood Glucose	Food Intake	Exercise

Medication   Symptoms   Notes
....
....
....
....
....

Date ....

Sleep quality and duration ....

Stress levels   1   2   3   4   5   6   7   8   9   10

Water Intake

Time	Blood Glucose	Food Intake	Exercise

Medication   Symptoms   Notes
....
....
....
....
....

Date ....

Sleep quality and duration ....

Stress levels   1   2   3   4   5   6   7   8   9   10

Water Intake   ▯ ▯ ▯ ▯ ▯ ▯ ▯ ▯ ▯ ▯

Time	Blood Glucose	Food Intake	Exercise

Medication   Symptoms   Notes
....
....
....
....
....

Date ....

Sleep quality and duration ....

Stress levels   1   2   3   4   5   6   7   8   9   10

Water Intake   ⌴ ⌴ ⌴ ⌴ ⌴ ⌴ ⌴ ⌴ ⌴ ⌴

Time	Blood Glucose	Food Intake	Exercise

Medication   Symptoms   Notes
....
....
....
....
....

Date ....

Sleep quality and duration ....

Stress levels   1   2   3   4   5   6   7   8   9   10

Water Intake

Time	Blood Glucose	Food Intake	Exercise

Medication   Symptoms   Notes

Date ....

Sleep quality and duration ....

Stress levels   1   2   3   4   5   6   7   8   9   10

Water Intake

Time	Blood Glucose	Food Intake	Exercise

Medication   Symptoms   Notes

Date ....

Sleep quality and duration ....

Stress levels   1   2   3   4   5   6   7   8   9   10

Water Intake   ▯   ▯   ▯   ▯   ▯   ▯   ▯   ▯   ▯   ▯

Time	Blood Glucose	Food Intake	Exercise

Medication   Symptoms   Notes
....
....
....
....
....

Date ....

Sleep quality and duration ....

Stress levels   1   2   3   4   5   6   7   8   9   10

Water Intake ▯ ▯ ▯ ▯ ▯ ▯ ▯ ▯ ▯ ▯

Time	Blood Glucose	Food Intake	Exercise

Medication   Symptoms   Notes
....
....
....
....
....

Date ....

Sleep quality and duration ....

Stress levels   1   2   3   4   5   6   7   8   9   10

Water Intake ⬜ ⬜ ⬜ ⬜ ⬜ ⬜ ⬜ ⬜ ⬜ ⬜

Time	Blood Glucose	Food Intake	Exercise

Medication   Symptoms   Notes
....
....
....
....
....

Date ....

Sleep quality and duration ....

Stress levels   1   2   3   4   5   6   7   8   9   10

Water Intake   ⬜ ⬜ ⬜ ⬜ ⬜ ⬜ ⬜ ⬜ ⬜ ⬜

Time	Blood Glucose	Food Intake	Exercise

Medication   Symptoms   Notes
....
....
....
....
....

Date ....

Sleep quality and duration ....

Stress levels   1   2   3   4   5   6   7   8   9   10

Water Intake   ▯ ▯ ▯ ▯ ▯ ▯ ▯ ▯ ▯ ▯

Time	Blood Glucose	Food Intake	Exercise

Medication   Symptoms   Notes
....
....
....
....
....

Date ....

Sleep quality and duration ....

Stress levels   1   2   3   4   5   6   7   8   9   10

Water Intake   ⬜ ⬜ ⬜ ⬜ ⬜ ⬜ ⬜ ⬜ ⬜ ⬜

Time	Blood Glucose	Food Intake	Exercise

Medication   Symptoms   Notes
....
....
....
....
....

Date ....

Sleep quality and duration ....

Stress levels   1   2   3   4   5   6   7   8   9   10

Water Intake   ▯ ▯ ▯ ▯ ▯ ▯ ▯ ▯ ▯ ▯

Time	Blood Glucose	Food Intake	Exercise

Medication   Symptoms   Notes
....
....
....
....
....

Date ....

Sleep quality and duration ....

Stress levels   1   2   3   4   5   6   7   8   9   10

Water Intake   ▢ ▢ ▢ ▢ ▢ ▢ ▢ ▢ ▢ ▢

Time	Blood Glucose	Food Intake	Exercise

Medication   Symptoms   Notes
....
....
....
....
....

Date ....

Sleep quality and duration ....

Stress levels   1   2   3   4   5   6   7   8   9   10

Water Intake   ▢ ▢ ▢ ▢ ▢ ▢ ▢ ▢ ▢ ▢

Time	Blood Glucose	Food Intake	Exercise

Medication   Symptoms   Notes
....
....
....
....
....

Date ....

Sleep quality and duration ....

Stress levels   1   2   3   4   5   6   7   8   9   10

Water Intake   ⌴ ⌴ ⌴ ⌴ ⌴ ⌴ ⌴ ⌴ ⌴ ⌴

Time	Blood Glucose	Food Intake	Exercise

Medication   Symptoms   Notes
....
....
....
....
....

Date ....

Sleep quality and duration ....

Stress levels   1   2   3   4   5   6   7   8   9   10

Water Intake   ▢ ▢ ▢ ▢ ▢ ▢ ▢ ▢ ▢ ▢

Time	Blood Glucose	Food Intake	Exercise

Medication   Symptoms   Notes
....
....
....
....
....

Date ....

Sleep quality and duration ....

Stress levels   1   2   3   4   5   6   7   8   9   10

Water Intake   ⊔ ⊔ ⊔ ⊔ ⊔ ⊔ ⊔ ⊔ ⊔ ⊔

Time	Blood Glucose	Food Intake	Exercise

Medication   Symptoms   Notes
....
....
....
....
....

Date ....

Sleep quality and duration ....

Stress levels　　1　2　3　4　5　6　7　8　9　10

Water Intake　▯ ▯ ▯ ▯ ▯ ▯ ▯ ▯ ▯ ▯

Time	Blood Glucose	Food Intake	Exercise

Medication　　　　　　Symptoms　　　　　　　Notes
....　..............................　..............................
....　..............................　..............................
....　..............................　..............................
....　..............................　..............................
....　..............................　..............................

Date ....

Sleep quality and duration ....

Stress levels   1   2   3   4   5   6   7   8   9   10

Water Intake

Time	Blood Glucose	Food Intake	Exercise

Medication   Symptoms   Notes

Date ....

Sleep quality and duration ....

Stress levels   1   2   3   4   5   6   7   8   9   10

Water Intake   ☐ ☐ ☐ ☐ ☐ ☐ ☐ ☐ ☐ ☐

Time	Blood Glucose	Food Intake	Exercise

Medication   Symptoms   Notes
....
....
....
....
....

Date ....

Sleep quality and duration ....

Stress levels   1   2   3   4   5   6   7   8   9   10

Water Intake   ▢ ▢ ▢ ▢ ▢ ▢ ▢ ▢ ▢ ▢

Time	Blood Glucose	Food Intake	Exercise

Medication   Symptoms   Notes
....
....
....
....
....

Date ....

Sleep quality and duration ....

Stress levels   1   2   3   4   5   6   7   8   9   10

Water Intake ⌤ ⌤ ⌤ ⌤ ⌤ ⌤ ⌤ ⌤ ⌤ ⌤

Time	Blood Glucose	Food Intake	Exercise

Medication   Symptoms   Notes
....
....
....
....
....

Date ....

Sleep quality and duration ....

Stress levels   1   2   3   4   5   6   7   8   9   10

Water Intake ⬜ ⬜ ⬜ ⬜ ⬜ ⬜ ⬜ ⬜ ⬜ ⬜

Time	Blood Glucose	Food Intake	Exercise

Medication   Symptoms   Notes
....
....
....
....
....

Date ....

Sleep quality and duration ....

Stress levels   1   2   3   4   5   6   7   8   9   10

Water Intake   ▭ ▭ ▭ ▭ ▭ ▭ ▭ ▭ ▭ ▭

Time	Blood Glucose	Food Intake	Exercise

Medication   Symptoms   Notes
....
....
....
....
....

Date ....

Sleep quality and duration ....

Stress levels   1   2   3   4   5   6   7   8   9   10

Water Intake ⎕ ⎕ ⎕ ⎕ ⎕ ⎕ ⎕ ⎕ ⎕ ⎕

Time	Blood Glucose	Food Intake	Exercise

Medication   Symptoms   Notes
....
....
....
....
....

Date ....

Sleep quality and duration ....

Stress levels   1   2   3   4   5   6   7   8   9   10

Water Intake   ▯ ▯ ▯ ▯ ▯ ▯ ▯ ▯ ▯ ▯

Time	Blood Glucose	Food Intake	Exercise

Medication   Symptoms   Notes
....
....
....
....
....

Date ....

Sleep quality and duration ....

Stress levels   1   2   3   4   5   6   7   8   9   10

Water Intake ▯ ▯ ▯ ▯ ▯ ▯ ▯ ▯ ▯ ▯

Time	Blood Glucose	Food Intake	Exercise

Medication   Symptoms   Notes
....
....
....
....
....

Date ....

Sleep quality and duration ....

Stress levels   1   2   3   4   5   6   7   8   9   10

Water Intake   ⎕ ⎕ ⎕ ⎕ ⎕ ⎕ ⎕ ⎕ ⎕ ⎕

Time	Blood Glucose	Food Intake	Exercise

Medication   Symptoms   Notes
....
....
....
....
....

Date ....

Sleep quality and duration ....

Stress levels   1   2   3   4   5   6   7   8   9   10

Water Intake

Time	Blood Glucose	Food Intake	Exercise

Medication   Symptoms   Notes
....
....
....
....
....

Date ....

Sleep quality and duration ....

Stress levels 1 2 3 4 5 6 7 8 9 10

Water Intake ⬜ ⬜ ⬜ ⬜ ⬜ ⬜ ⬜ ⬜ ⬜ ⬜

Time	Blood Glucose	Food Intake	Exercise

Medication   Symptoms   Notes
....
....
....
....
....

Date ....

Sleep quality and duration ....

Stress levels   1   2   3   4   5   6   7   8   9   10

Water Intake ⬜ ⬜ ⬜ ⬜ ⬜ ⬜ ⬜ ⬜ ⬜ ⬜

Time	Blood Glucose	Food Intake	Exercise

Medication   Symptoms   Notes
....
....
....
....
....

Date ....

Sleep quality and duration ....

Stress levels   1   2   3   4   5   6   7   8   9   10

Water Intake   ▯   ▯   ▯   ▯   ▯   ▯   ▯   ▯   ▯   ▯

Time	Blood Glucose	Food Intake	Exercise

Medication   Symptoms   Notes
....
....
....
....
....

Date ....

Sleep quality and duration ....

Stress levels   1   2   3   4   5   6   7   8   9   10

Water Intake ▯ ▯ ▯ ▯ ▯ ▯ ▯ ▯ ▯ ▯

Time	Blood Glucose	Food Intake	Exercise

Medication   Symptoms   Notes
....
....
....
....
....

Date ....

Sleep quality and duration ....

Stress levels   1   2   3   4   5   6   7   8   9   10

Water Intake ▯ ▯ ▯ ▯ ▯ ▯ ▯ ▯ ▯ ▯

Time	Blood Glucose	Food Intake	Exercise

Medication   Symptoms   Notes
....
....
....
....
....

Date ....

Sleep quality and duration ....

Stress levels   1   2   3   4   5   6   7   8   9   10

Water Intake ⬜ ⬜ ⬜ ⬜ ⬜ ⬜ ⬜ ⬜ ⬜ ⬜

Time	Blood Glucose	Food Intake	Exercise

Medication   Symptoms   Notes
....
....
....
....
....

Date ....

Sleep quality and duration ....

Stress levels   1   2   3   4   5   6   7   8   9   10

Water Intake ⌴ ⌴ ⌴ ⌴ ⌴ ⌴ ⌴ ⌴ ⌴ ⌴

Time	Blood Glucose	Food Intake	Exercise

Medication   Symptoms   Notes
....
....
....
....
....

Date ....

Sleep quality and duration ....

Stress levels   1   2   3   4   5   6   7   8   9   10

Water Intake   ▢ ▢ ▢ ▢ ▢ ▢ ▢ ▢ ▢ ▢

Time	Blood Glucose	Food Intake	Exercise

Medication   Symptoms   Notes

....

....

....

....

....

Date ....

Sleep quality and duration ....

Stress levels   1   2   3   4   5   6   7   8   9   10

Water Intake   ▢ ▢ ▢ ▢ ▢ ▢ ▢ ▢ ▢ ▢

Time	Blood Glucose	Food Intake	Exercise

Medication   Symptoms   Notes
....
....
....
....
....

Date ....

Sleep quality and duration ....

Stress levels   1   2   3   4   5   6   7   8   9   10

Water Intake ▯ ▯ ▯ ▯ ▯ ▯ ▯ ▯ ▯ ▯

Time	Blood Glucose	Food Intake	Exercise

Medication   Symptoms   Notes
....
....
....
....
....

Date ....

Sleep quality and duration ....

Stress levels   1   2   3   4   5   6   7   8   9   10

Water Intake   ☐ ☐ ☐ ☐ ☐ ☐ ☐ ☐ ☐ ☐

Time	Blood Glucose	Food Intake	Exercise

Medication   Symptoms   Notes
....
....
....
....
....

Date ....

Sleep quality and duration ....

Stress levels   1   2   3   4   5   6   7   8   9   10

Water Intake ▯ ▯ ▯ ▯ ▯ ▯ ▯ ▯ ▯ ▯

Time	Blood Glucose	Food Intake	Exercise

Medication   Symptoms   Notes
....
....
....
....
....

Date ....

Sleep quality and duration ....

Stress levels   1   2   3   4   5   6   7   8   9   10

Water Intake

Time	Blood Glucose	Food Intake	Exercise

Medication   Symptoms   Notes
....
....
....
....
....

Date ....

Sleep quality and duration ....

Stress levels   1   2   3   4   5   6   7   8   9   10

Water Intake   ⬜ ⬜ ⬜ ⬜ ⬜ ⬜ ⬜ ⬜ ⬜ ⬜

Time	Blood Glucose	Food Intake	Exercise

Medication   Symptoms   Notes
....
....
....
....
....

Date ....

Sleep quality and duration ....

Stress levels   1   2   3   4   5   6   7   8   9   10

Water Intake   ⌄ ⌄ ⌄ ⌄ ⌄ ⌄ ⌄ ⌄ ⌄ ⌄

Time	Blood Glucose	Food Intake	Exercise

Medication   Symptoms   Notes
....
....
....
....
....

Date ....

Sleep quality and duration ....

Stress levels   1   2   3   4   5   6   7   8   9   10

Water Intake   ▯ ▯ ▯ ▯ ▯ ▯ ▯ ▯ ▯ ▯

Time	Blood Glucose	Food Intake	Exercise

Medication	Symptoms	Notes
....	....	....
....	....	....
....	....	....
....	....	....
....	....	....

Date ....

Sleep quality and duration ....

Stress levels   1   2   3   4   5   6   7   8   9   10

Water Intake   ☐ ☐ ☐ ☐ ☐ ☐ ☐ ☐ ☐ ☐

Time	Blood Glucose	Food Intake	Exercise

Medication   Symptoms   Notes
....
....
....
....
....

Date ....

Sleep quality and duration ....

Stress levels   1   2   3   4   5   6   7   8   9   10

Water Intake

Time	Blood Glucose	Food Intake	Exercise

Medication   Symptoms   Notes
....
....
....
....
....

Date ....

Sleep quality and duration ....

Stress levels   1   2   3   4   5   6   7   8   9   10

Water Intake   ▯ ▯ ▯ ▯ ▯ ▯ ▯ ▯ ▯ ▯

Time	Blood Glucose	Food Intake	Exercise

Medication   Symptoms   Notes

....

....

....

....

....

Date ....

Sleep quality and duration ....

Stress levels   1   2   3   4   5   6   7   8   9   10

Water Intake

Time	Blood Glucose	Food Intake	Exercise

Medication   Symptoms   Notes

Date ....

Sleep quality and duration ....

Stress levels   1   2   3   4   5   6   7   8   9   10

Water Intake   ▢ ▢ ▢ ▢ ▢ ▢ ▢ ▢ ▢ ▢

Time	Blood Glucose	Food Intake	Exercise

Medication   Symptoms   Notes
....
....
....
....
....

Date ....

Sleep quality and duration ....

Stress levels   1   2   3   4   5   6   7   8   9   10

Water Intake ▢ ▢ ▢ ▢ ▢ ▢ ▢ ▢ ▢ ▢

Time	Blood Glucose	Food Intake	Exercise

Medication   Symptoms   Notes
....
....
....
....
....

Date ....

Sleep quality and duration ....

Stress levels   1   2   3   4   5   6   7   8   9   10

Water Intake   ☐ ☐ ☐ ☐ ☐ ☐ ☐ ☐ ☐ ☐

Time	Blood Glucose	Food Intake	Exercise

Medication   Symptoms   Notes

Date ....

Sleep quality and duration ....

Stress levels   1   2   3   4   5   6   7   8   9   10

Water Intake   ▢ ▢ ▢ ▢ ▢ ▢ ▢ ▢ ▢ ▢

Time	Blood Glucose	Food Intake	Exercise

Medication   Symptoms   Notes
....
....
....
....
....

Date ....

Sleep quality and duration ....

Stress levels   1   2   3   4   5   6   7   8   9   10

Water Intake   ▢ ▢ ▢ ▢ ▢ ▢ ▢ ▢ ▢ ▢

Time	Blood Glucose	Food Intake	Exercise

Medication   Symptoms   Notes
....
....
....
....
....

Date ....

Sleep quality and duration ....

Stress levels   1   2   3   4   5   6   7   8   9   10

Water Intake   ⬜ ⬜ ⬜ ⬜ ⬜ ⬜ ⬜ ⬜ ⬜ ⬜

Time	Blood Glucose	Food Intake	Exercise

Medication   Symptoms   Notes
....
....
....
....
....

Date ....

Sleep quality and duration ....

Stress levels   1   2   3   4   5   6   7   8   9   10

Water Intake ▯ ▯ ▯ ▯ ▯ ▯ ▯ ▯ ▯ ▯

Time	Blood Glucose	Food Intake	Exercise

Medication   Symptoms   Notes
....
....
....
....
....

Date ....

Sleep quality and duration ....

Stress levels   1   2   3   4   5   6   7   8   9   10

Water Intake   ▯ ▯ ▯ ▯ ▯ ▯ ▯ ▯ ▯ ▯

Time	Blood Glucose	Food Intake	Exercise

Medication   Symptoms   Notes
....
....
....
....
....

Date ....

Sleep quality and duration ....

Stress levels   1   2   3   4   5   6   7   8   9   10

Water Intake ▢ ▢ ▢ ▢ ▢ ▢ ▢ ▢ ▢ ▢

Time	Blood Glucose	Food Intake	Exercise

Medication   Symptoms   Notes
....
....
....
....
....

Date ....

Sleep quality and duration ....

Stress levels   1   2   3   4   5   6   7   8   9   10

Water Intake   ▯ ▯ ▯ ▯ ▯ ▯ ▯ ▯ ▯ ▯

Time	Blood Glucose	Food Intake	Exercise

Medication   Symptoms   Notes
....
....
....
....
....

Date ....

Sleep quality and duration ....

Stress levels   1   2   3   4   5   6   7   8   9   10

Water Intake   ☐ ☐ ☐ ☐ ☐ ☐ ☐ ☐ ☐ ☐

Time	Blood Glucose	Food Intake	Exercise

Medication   Symptoms   Notes
....
....
....
....
....

Date ....

Sleep quality and duration ....

Stress levels   1   2   3   4   5   6   7   8   9   10

Water Intake   ☐ ☐ ☐ ☐ ☐ ☐ ☐ ☐ ☐ ☐

Time	Blood Glucose	Food Intake	Exercise

Medication   Symptoms   Notes
....
....
....
....
....

Date ....

Sleep quality and duration ....

Stress levels   1   2   3   4   5   6   7   8   9   10

Water Intake ⬜ ⬜ ⬜ ⬜ ⬜ ⬜ ⬜ ⬜ ⬜ ⬜

Time	Blood Glucose	Food Intake	Exercise

Medication   Symptoms   Notes
....
....
....
....
....

Date ....

Sleep quality and duration ....

Stress levels   1   2   3   4   5   6   7   8   9   10

Water Intake   ⊔ ⊔ ⊔ ⊔ ⊔ ⊔ ⊔ ⊔ ⊔ ⊔

Time	Blood Glucose	Food Intake	Exercise

Medication   Symptoms   Notes
....
....
....
....
....

Date ....

Sleep quality and duration ....

Stress levels   1   2   3   4   5   6   7   8   9   10

Water Intake   ☐ ☐ ☐ ☐ ☐ ☐ ☐ ☐ ☐ ☐

Time	Blood Glucose	Food Intake	Exercise

Medication   Symptoms   Notes
....
....
....
....
....

Date ....

Sleep quality and duration ....

Stress levels   1   2   3   4   5   6   7   8   9   10

Water Intake   ▢ ▢ ▢ ▢ ▢ ▢ ▢ ▢ ▢ ▢

Time	Blood Glucose	Food Intake	Exercise

Medication   Symptoms   Notes
....
....
....
....
....

Date ....

Sleep quality and duration ....

Stress levels   1   2   3   4   5   6   7   8   9   10

Water Intake   ▢ ▢ ▢ ▢ ▢ ▢ ▢ ▢ ▢ ▢

Time	Blood Glucose	Food Intake	Exercise

Medication   Symptoms   Notes
....
....
....
....
....

Date ....

Sleep quality and duration ....

Stress levels   1   2   3   4   5   6   7   8   9   10

Water Intake   ▢ ▢ ▢ ▢ ▢ ▢ ▢ ▢ ▢ ▢

Time	Blood Glucose	Food Intake	Exercise

Medication   Symptoms   Notes
....
....
....
....
....

Date ....

Sleep quality and duration ....

Stress levels   1   2   3   4   5   6   7   8   9   10

Water Intake   ⬜ ⬜ ⬜ ⬜ ⬜ ⬜ ⬜ ⬜ ⬜ ⬜

Time	Blood Glucose	Food Intake	Exercise

Medication   Symptoms   Notes
....
....
....
....
....

Date ....

Sleep quality and duration ....

Stress levels   1   2   3   4   5   6   7   8   9   10

Water Intake   ▯ ▯ ▯ ▯ ▯ ▯ ▯ ▯ ▯ ▯

Time	Blood Glucose	Food Intake	Exercise

Medication   Symptoms   Notes
....
....
....
....
....

Date ....

Sleep quality and duration ....

Stress levels   1   2   3   4   5   6   7   8   9   10

Water Intake

Time	Blood Glucose	Food Intake	Exercise

Medication   Symptoms   Notes

Date ....

Sleep quality and duration ....

Stress levels   1   2   3   4   5   6   7   8   9   10

Water Intake   ▢ ▢ ▢ ▢ ▢ ▢ ▢ ▢ ▢ ▢

Time	Blood Glucose	Food Intake	Exercise

Medication   Symptoms   Notes
....
....
....
....
....

Date ....

Sleep quality and duration ....

Stress levels   1   2   3   4   5   6   7   8   9   10

Water Intake   ▯ ▯ ▯ ▯ ▯ ▯ ▯ ▯ ▯ ▯

Time	Blood Glucose	Food Intake	Exercise

Medication   Symptoms   Notes
....
....
....
....
....

Date ....

Sleep quality and duration ....

Stress levels 1 2 3 4 5 6 7 8 9 10

Water Intake ☐ ☐ ☐ ☐ ☐ ☐ ☐ ☐ ☐ ☐

Time	Blood Glucose	Food Intake	Exercise

Medication   Symptoms   Notes
....
....
....
....
....

Date ....

Sleep quality and duration ....

Stress levels   1   2   3   4   5   6   7   8   9   10

Water Intake

Time	Blood Glucose	Food Intake	Exercise

Medication   Symptoms   Notes

Date ....

Sleep quality and duration ....

Stress levels   1   2   3   4   5   6   7   8   9   10

Water Intake   ⌴ ⌴ ⌴ ⌴ ⌴ ⌴ ⌴ ⌴ ⌴ ⌴

Time	Blood Glucose	Food Intake	Exercise

Medication   Symptoms   Notes
....
....
....
....
....

Date ....

Sleep quality and duration ....

Stress levels   1   2   3   4   5   6   7   8   9   10

Water Intake   ▯ ▯ ▯ ▯ ▯ ▯ ▯ ▯ ▯ ▯

Time	Blood Glucose	Food Intake	Exercise

Medication   Symptoms   Notes
....
....
....
....
....

Date ....

Sleep quality and duration ....

Stress levels   1   2   3   4   5   6   7   8   9   10

Water Intake   ☐ ☐ ☐ ☐ ☐ ☐ ☐ ☐ ☐ ☐

Time	Blood Glucose	Food Intake	Exercise

Medication   Symptoms   Notes
....
....
....
....
....

Date ....

Sleep quality and duration ....

Stress levels   1   2   3   4   5   6   7   8   9   10

Water Intake   ⬜ ⬜ ⬜ ⬜ ⬜ ⬜ ⬜ ⬜ ⬜ ⬜

Time	Blood Glucose	Food Intake	Exercise

Medication   Symptoms   Notes
....
....
....
....
....

Date ....

Sleep quality and duration ....

Stress levels   1   2   3   4   5   6   7   8   9   10

Water Intake   ▢ ▢ ▢ ▢ ▢ ▢ ▢ ▢ ▢ ▢

Time	Blood Glucose	Food Intake	Exercise

Medication   Symptoms   Notes
....
....
....
....
....

Date ....

Sleep quality and duration ....

Stress levels   1   2   3   4   5   6   7   8   9   10

Water Intake ⌴ ⌴ ⌴ ⌴ ⌴ ⌴ ⌴ ⌴ ⌴ ⌴

Time	Blood Glucose	Food Intake	Exercise

Medication   Symptoms   Notes
....
....
....
....
....

Date ....

Sleep quality and duration ....

Stress levels   1   2   3   4   5   6   7   8   9   10

Water Intake   ☐ ☐ ☐ ☐ ☐ ☐ ☐ ☐ ☐ ☐

Time	Blood Glucose	Food Intake	Exercise

Medication   Symptoms   Notes
....
....
....
....
....

Date ....

Sleep quality and duration ....

Stress levels   1   2   3   4   5   6   7   8   9   10

Water Intake   ▢ ▢ ▢ ▢ ▢ ▢ ▢ ▢ ▢ ▢

Time	Blood Glucose	Food Intake	Exercise

Medication   Symptoms   Notes
....
....
....
....
....

Date ....

Sleep quality and duration ....

Stress levels   1   2   3   4   5   6   7   8   9   10

Water Intake ▯ ▯ ▯ ▯ ▯ ▯ ▯ ▯ ▯ ▯

Time	Blood Glucose	Food Intake	Exercise

Medication   Symptoms   Notes
....
....
....
....
....

Date ....

Sleep quality and duration ....

Stress levels   1   2   3   4   5   6   7   8   9   10

Water Intake   ▢ ▢ ▢ ▢ ▢ ▢ ▢ ▢ ▢ ▢

Time	Blood Glucose	Food Intake	Exercise

Medication   Symptoms   Notes
....
....
....
....
....

Date ....

Sleep quality and duration ....

Stress levels   1   2   3   4   5   6   7   8   9   10

Water Intake ⌴ ⌴ ⌴ ⌴ ⌴ ⌴ ⌴ ⌴ ⌴ ⌴

Time	Blood Glucose	Food Intake	Exercise

Medication   Symptoms   Notes
....
....
....
....
....

Date ....

Sleep quality and duration ....

Stress levels   1   2   3   4   5   6   7   8   9   10

Water Intake   ▢ ▢ ▢ ▢ ▢ ▢ ▢ ▢ ▢ ▢

Time	Blood Glucose	Food Intake	Exercise

Medication   Symptoms   Notes
....
....
....
....
....

Date ....

Sleep quality and duration ....

Stress levels   1   2   3   4   5   6   7   8   9   10

Water Intake

Time	Blood Glucose	Food Intake	Exercise

Medication   Symptoms   Notes

Date ....

Sleep quality and duration ....

Stress levels   1   2   3   4   5   6   7   8   9   10

Water Intake ▯ ▯ ▯ ▯ ▯ ▯ ▯ ▯ ▯ ▯

Time	Blood Glucose	Food Intake	Exercise

Medication   Symptoms   Notes
....
....
....
....
....

Date ....

Sleep quality and duration ....

Stress levels   1   2   3   4   5   6   7   8   9   10

Water Intake   ☐ ☐ ☐ ☐ ☐ ☐ ☐ ☐ ☐ ☐

Time	Blood Glucose	Food Intake	Exercise

Medication   Symptoms   Notes
....
....
....
....
....

Date ....

Sleep quality and duration ....

Stress levels   1   2   3   4   5   6   7   8   9   10

Water Intake   ⬜ ⬜ ⬜ ⬜ ⬜ ⬜ ⬜ ⬜ ⬜ ⬜

Time	Blood Glucose	Food Intake	Exercise

Medication   Symptoms   Notes
....
....
....
....
....

Date ....

Sleep quality and duration ....

Stress levels   1   2   3   4   5   6   7   8   9   10

Water Intake ▯ ▯ ▯ ▯ ▯ ▯ ▯ ▯ ▯ ▯

Time	Blood Glucose	Food Intake	Exercise

Medication   Symptoms   Notes
....
....
....
....
....

Date ....

Sleep quality and duration ....

Stress levels   1   2   3   4   5   6   7   8   9   10

Water Intake ▯ ▯ ▯ ▯ ▯ ▯ ▯ ▯ ▯ ▯

Time	Blood Glucose	Food Intake	Exercise

Medication   Symptoms   Notes
....
....
....
....
....

Date ....

Sleep quality and duration ....

Stress levels   1   2   3   4   5   6   7   8   9   10

Water Intake   ⬜ ⬜ ⬜ ⬜ ⬜ ⬜ ⬜ ⬜ ⬜ ⬜

Time	Blood Glucose	Food Intake	Exercise

Medication   Symptoms   Notes
....
....
....
....
....

Date ....

Sleep quality and duration ....

Stress levels   1   2   3   4   5   6   7   8   9   10

Water Intake ⬜ ⬜ ⬜ ⬜ ⬜ ⬜ ⬜ ⬜ ⬜ ⬜

Time	Blood Glucose	Food Intake	Exercise

Medication   Symptoms   Notes
....
....
....
....
....

Date ....

Sleep quality and duration ....

Stress levels   1   2   3   4   5   6   7   8   9   10

Water Intake ☐ ☐ ☐ ☐ ☐ ☐ ☐ ☐ ☐ ☐

Time	Blood Glucose	Food Intake	Exercise

Medication	Symptoms	Notes
....	....	....
....	....	....
....	....	....
....	....	....
....	....	....

Date ....

Sleep quality and duration ....

Stress levels   1   2   3   4   5   6   7   8   9   10

Water Intake ⬜ ⬜ ⬜ ⬜ ⬜ ⬜ ⬜ ⬜ ⬜ ⬜

Time	Blood Glucose	Food Intake	Exercise

Medication   Symptoms   Notes
....
....
....
....
....

Date ....

Sleep quality and duration ....

Stress levels   1   2   3   4   5   6   7   8   9   10

Water Intake   ▢ ▢ ▢ ▢ ▢ ▢ ▢ ▢ ▢ ▢

Time	Blood Glucose	Food Intake	Exercise

Medication   Symptoms   Notes
....
....
....
....
....

Date ....

Sleep quality and duration ....

Stress levels   1   2   3   4   5   6   7   8   9   10

Water Intake ▯ ▯ ▯ ▯ ▯ ▯ ▯ ▯ ▯ ▯

Time	Blood Glucose	Food Intake	Exercise

Medication   Symptoms   Notes
....
....
....
....
....

Date ....

Sleep quality and duration ....

Stress levels   1   2   3   4   5   6   7   8   9   10

Water Intake

Time	Blood Glucose	Food Intake	Exercise

Medication   Symptoms   Notes
....
....
....
....
....

Made in the USA
Columbia, SC
09 December 2023